HEART ATTACK
(Mine . . . and Yours?)

HEART ATTACK
(Mine ... and Yours?)

Kenneth E. Geary

Exposition Press   **Hicksville, New York**

First Edition

© 1979 by Kenneth E. Geary

ISBN 0-682-49348-1

Printed in the United States of America

To my wife, JoAnn,
without whose presence of mind
in a time of emergency
there would be no tomorrows

CONTENTS

FOREWORD

Each day there will be hundreds of men and women who will experience the pain and fright known as heart attack. Some, a minority, will not survive. For those more fortunate, life will go on but will not be quite the same again. The knowledge of one's heart disease now exists. Recurring symptoms must be greeted and new plans must be laid for the future. What's it like? Where does one turn when this intrusion has forced its way in? Kenneth Geary has been through it, and very ably tells his story. It will be of benefit to those who for one reason or another have an interest in coronary heart disease or who, perhaps, simply have an interest in human survival.

A. ERIK GUNDERSEN, M.D.
Chief, Cardiac Surgery
Gundersen Clinic, Ltd.
La Crosse, Wisconsin

HEART ATTACK
(Mine . . . and Yours?)

INTRODUCTION

So you had a heart attack! Well, so did I, and I guess that gives us enough in common so that we can take a few minutes of each other's time and share our experiences— yours with me through your thoughts as you read and mine with you as I attempt to convey the events that immediately preceded my heart attack, my fleeting remembrance of the things that happened during it, and the multitude of things that happened after, including my open-heart surgery, rehabilitation, and subsequent return to work responsibilities.

Perhaps many of the things I relate will strike a familiar chord in terms of your heart attack, or perhaps they will present a side that is completely different; but regardless of the similarity or dissimilarity of the date, time, and occurrence, we all will agree on one thing—once is enough! The degree of severity of the attacks, although important, is not the overriding factor; what is is the fact that the next time we may not be fortunate enough to remember, and, speaking of remembering, I like to think that you and I, and the thousands of men and women that have had and who will have similar experiences in their lifetime, are unique, special people. We have to be because we have come so close to the last scene in life and yet the final curtain was held back; we were given a repieve—an extension of time if you will—hopefully for a special reason.

My wife, except for whose actions I would not have made it through the initial stages of my attack, has told me many times that the good Lord must have been watching over me during this time, and I like to believe that she is right, not only for me but for you, too; and if he was, he must have had a reason for doing so. Let's try and find out what that reason was and is. This time around may be our last, so let's make it the best!

Good luck, get better soon, keep up the exercises, watch the diet, and may God continue to bless you in every way possible.

PROLOGUE TO
A HEART ATTACK

My daughter, Lisa, had an orthodontist appointment in La Crosse, Wisconsin, scheduled for the morning of June 19, 1975, and I had made arrangements to have the day off from my work responsibilities so that our entire family might visit relatives in that city and shop before and after Lisa's dental appointment. My wife and I had awakened early and at approximately eight o'clock were making every effort to have our daughter and our two sons hurry so that we might depart as early as possible. As June 19 fell on a Thursday, it was also the designated day for collection of rubbish and garbage from our neighborhood, and, as our containers were not yet at the curb side, I left the house to accommodate this task.

Please understand that at this time and for all my time prior to this moment, I had never had, nor did I think I could have, any problem associated with my heart or my circulatory system—or any other system as far as that goes. I was forty-six years old, weighed approximately one hundred and fifty pounds, was six feet tall, smoked a package and a half of cigarettes a day (sometimes more), enjoyed a glass of beer occasionally, had never been in a hospital for a personal illness or surgical procedure (except for a stitched lip from a childhood fight), enjoyed the outdoors and hunting and fishing as much if not more than the "other" fellow, and, for all practical purposes, felt that I would live to be at least one hundred years of age. After all, my dad always said that it took a lean horse to run a long race, and I was certainly in the "lean" category.

I had attended a teacher training institution after graduation from high school, and, after receiving my initial degree and serving my two years in the armed forces during the Korean War, began my career in the teaching profession in 1954. During the next twenty odd years up to the day of my attack, I enjoyed my work and the feeling of contribution associated with it. My wife Joan was also a teacher, and during the time preceding my heart attack was volunteering her professional expertise in the field of Library Science by assisting in the Instructional Materials Center of the St. Peter and Paul Parochial School in our community. Our children, to whom I alluded briefly before, number three and include our daughter, Lisa, age fourteen at the time of my heart attack, and our twin sons, Ted and Todd, who were twelve at the time. All in all, my life was very satisfying, things were going well, my family enjoyed good health, and we were looking forward to a day of shopping and visiting.

It was a clear, beautiful, cool day, and I can remember as plainly as yesterday leaving the house to carry the garbage cans to the curb. The distance from the back of our garage where the containers are located to the curb is about thirty-five yards, and I made the trip back and forth a total of four times, three times carrying a container and the fourth time wheeling a wheelbarrow. At no time during this limited exertion did I feel any pains in my chest or any tingling sensation in my arms or other extremities; nor did I experience to the best of my recollection any shortness of breath, as one normally would during heavy exertion. After finishing this task, I began to walk back to the house to wash up prior to leaving, and it was at this time, while I was still outside, that I began to perspire and feel an overwhelming weakness that continued with me and became progressively more pronounced as I entered the house.

I remember my wife asking me if anything was wrong and my profound answer that I didn't know; but I thought that if I sat down for a moment, my tired and overheated condition would go away. How wrong I was! When I say that the feeling I have described became progressively worse, I can best convey this by indicating to you that a few moments of sitting in a chair did nothing to relieve the feeling I was experiencing. I became warmer and warmer along with a weakening condition that internally cried out for rest. I do not recall the specific items of clothing that I was wearing at this time, but I do recall saying, if not to someone then to myself, that I had to lie down for a while; and because I was so warm, I had to take off some of my clothing. The final thing I remember about this stage of my heart attack was struggling to take off one item of clothing after another as I lay on the bed, and then I must have, at least temporarily, lost consciousness.

My wife has indicated to me the concurrent events of our household at this time, and she has related to me that one of the parish board members of our church had called at our home during the time I was sitting on the dining room chair, trying to relax and overcome my tiredness, and he had asked if I could visit the church parsonage kitchen with him about a matter concerning the remodeling of same. After my wife had told him that we were leaving shortly for La Crosse for our daughter's dental appointment and that I was not feeling well, she returned to the dining room of our home to find that I had gone to the bedroom and was there trying to take my clothing off, while at the same time rolling in an uneasy fashion from side to side on the bed. It was at this time that she took my pulse, and, even though she found my pulse normal, telephoned for an ambulance to pick me up. Then she immediately called the nearest hospital at Whitehall, Wisconsin (five miles east of our home) to make sure a doctor would be available when we arrived.

I can recall hearing my wife talking on the telephone about someone being sick and about an ambulance being necessary, but only in bits and pieces. When I reflect on the fact that my wife called an ambulance at this time, even after taking my pulse and finding it normal, I am gratified at what I must call her intuition. I have thought about this often, and have wondered if I would have done the same thing or reacted in the same way if our positions had been reversed. I honestly feel that I may have prolonged calling an ambulance in the hope that the situation would improve. Thank God she didn't—it surely would have proven fatal to me!

I do not know how long it was from the time my wife initially called until the ambulance arrived. She has since told me that it seemed forever, but was actually about ten minutes. I do know that the next thing I recalled was the presence of people in my bedroom, and these people were getting me out of bed onto a stretcher and wheeling me out of the house through the living room, out the front door, and into a waiting vehicle. The only person I could identify at this time was the chief of police of our community, who had arrived to assist in any way possible. For some reason, it felt good to have him there. The only thing I can remember about the ambulance ride to the hospital was someone's conversation with the hospital that the ambulance's ETA was approximately four to five minutes. That was the last thing I remembered about the ambulance ride.

When I reflect on my heart attack from incidence to the moment of being transported to the Whitehall hospital, the strangest thing of all to me is the fact that not once during this time did I experience any pain associated with the attack—only the feeling of warmth and tiredness that I described earlier and then apparent unconsciousness or partial unconsciousness. I can recall thinking that if this was what it was like to die, how easy it must be!

TRANSFER TO
INTENSIVE CARE

Have you ever had a dream in which you were about to be attacked or harmed, and just as you raised your arms in defense of the impending danger, you awakened? This is the best way that I can describe my next recollection of what I was experiencing. Although I do not recall arriving at the Whitehall Hospital, I do vividly remember that I was lying on a hard table or bench and that someone was pounding on my chest with such a force that I thought my ribs would surely break. The pain was excruciating and in an effort to stop whoever was administering this punishment, I raised my arms in a feeble attempt to make him stop. This is all I can remember about my brief stop at the Whitehall Memorial Hospital, although I have since been told that I was very fortunate in that when I arrived in the ambulance, there was present at the hospital a consulting physician from Winona, Minnesota, who had extensive training and experience in dealing with heart attack patients. This doctor and a regular Whitehall Hospital staff physician both worked on me to maintain a heartbeat, which to say the least was fragile. It was at this time that one of the attending physicians contacted the Lutheran Hospital in La Crosse and arranged for a cardiac ambulance to transfer me to that institution immediately for follow-up care. It was after this call had been made and while I was still in an apparently stable condition that my heart went into a condition called "fribulation"—a wild, uncontrolled rhythm of the heart that, if unchecked, could result in death. It was at this point that the visiting physician I referred to earlier arrested the fribulation by administering the sharp blows to my chest and heart. Can you imagine me trying to stop him? He undoubtedly saved my life, for which I will be eternally grateful. It is interesting to note that since my recovery, I have been told by the regular staff physician who assisted me that evening that he never thought I would survive the trip to La Crosse in the ambulance! I must have been a pretty picture!

The only thing that I can remember about the ride in the cardiac ambulance from Whitehall, Wisconsin, to the Lutheran Hospital in La Crosse, Wisconsin—a distance of approximately forty-five miles—is a vague recollection that someone in the ambulance was radioing ahead that he needed some type of medication and the return response that the ambulance was to stop in Holmen, Wisconsin, to pick up the required medication. The next thing I remember was awakening in the cardiac care unit of the La Crosse Lutheran Hospital, where I was adorned with not only the nuts and bolts necessary to monitor a human heart and to report its every movement, but also with the equipment necessary to allow the body to carry on its life functions without the necessity of the slightest exertion.

I remained in the cardiac care unit of the La Crosse Lutheran Hospital from June 19 until June 30, 1975, and as I look back now on the events of those ten days, it is more difficult to recall the specific events than the total care. I do recall that one of the first things I noticed about my hardware adornment was the fact that a pacemaker had been inserted into my heart from the shoulder area, and when I inquired about this I was told that immediately after I had arrived from Whitehall, my heart had again gone into fribulation and the doctors in attendance had a difficult time stabilizing my condition. The insertion of the pacemaker was to prevent such a recurrence, and it would remain in place until the doctors felt certain that fribulation would not occur again.

In addition to the pacemaker, the initial days in cardiac care saw me adorned with intravenous feeding tubes, electrocardiogram connections, breathing attachments, and related items thought necessary to maintain and enhance a stable and strengthening condition. As I indicated earlier, the main impression that I recall from this phase of my hospitalization was the wonderful care that was given me by those in attendance. I sincerely believe, and I hope you do too, that the positive comments and reassurance of well-being that these people extend to their patients contribute greatly to a person's speedy recovery; I know it did for me, and at this point I would like to say a special word of thanks to all the thousands, nay millions, of men and women who have dedicated their lives to the profession of caring for the sick and maimed, regardless of walk of life. If you, the reader, have experienced the need for intensive care under any circumstances, I sincerely hope that your care was equal to mine—because if it was, you had the finest possible. Never could I find the words to express to the men and women who were charged with the responsibility of my care, my deep and honest love for their tenderness and compassion, which they not only expressed through their oral responses to my needs, but also through their excellent professional care. If the physical impairment of a heart attack must of necessity be treated with a precise science and physical means, so I am convinced that the psychological despair that I experienced those first days in that cardiac care unit can be treated only with a genuine care and empathy that together can make a spirit rise and self-respect return. The feeling of helplessness and total dependency can be debilitating, and if you have experienced this, you know what I mean. Thanks again to those who go beyond themselves to help the likes of us back to reality and daily living.

After untold X rays, blood counts, urine analysis tests, inhalation therapy exercises, glucose feedings, and words of encouragement, and after daily showings of improvement and increased strength resulting in the luxury of being able to sit in a chair and walk a few steps, the pacemaker was removed, the wires and tubes disappeared, and feeding became a routine matter completed by a simple process learned in infancy and perfected in early childhood—the use of one's own hands. It was June 30, 1975, and I was transferred to a regular room on the third floor of the hospital.

The remaining days of my initial stay at the hospital were primarily devoted to watchful care and daily strengthening and improvement enhanced by routine exercise. On the second full day of "regular room" care, I was introduced to a modified graded exercise test, a GXT. I can remember being wheeled to a different section of the hospital and upon arriving at the location, being asked to lie upon a table where the attendants proceeded to apply the connectors from the electrocardiograph machine to my chest with long leads, which would allow me freedom to stand erect and to simulate walking on a continuous treadmill. The treadmill could be automatically adjusted by the doctor in charge to whatever plane or whatever speed he desired. If you have had the experience of taking this test, you know that it can be quite exhausting, and it was no different with me, for at certain stages of the test, breathing became quite difficult as I am sure it was intended to be. In addition, my legs became quite tired and I was not disappointed in the least when the test was concluded. Those in attendance seemed to feel that the results were good, however, and this did wonders for my feeling of well-being. After returning to my room, I was feeling quite good about my total progress and looking forward to the day, hopefully before the Fourth of July, when I could return home. However, the Fourth of July was to see a reduction in hospital staff for the holiday, and because of this certain tests, which were deemed necessary to make a final prognosis of my overall condition, were postponed. Subsequently, my release from the hospital was postponed and my observance of this holiday was made from my hospital room rather than my home. My family was with me, however, and it was only a matter of a few days before I would be discharged.

The days that followed were routine hospitalization days with routine activities such as blood pressure checks, blood tests, administration of medication (I was taking Quinidine and Quinaglute at this time), and continuing exercise. Then, on July 9, I had the pleasure of participating in what I consider to be the most uncomfortable tests (if you have had them I know you will agree) that I experienced during my entire stay in the hospital—a right and left catheterization of the heart and a coronary angiography. Before you begin to believe that this is an excruciatingly painful test, let me hasten to reassure you that it is not painful in any sense of the word. In the test referred to, I was placed on a sophisticated table contoured to fit the roundness of the body and then strapped securely on same so that there would be absolutely no movement of the body or head. The table itself was capable of being adjusted to any angle or plane, vertical or horizontal, or of being completely inverted if such was the desire. It is my understanding that a catheter or small tube is inserted into the groin area and thence into the main vein leading to the heart. This tube is then threaded with infinite care and skill to the heart, the physician in charge being able to view the progress of the catheter through the vein on an X-ray monitor screen. I was wide awake during this procedure and could catch glimpses of the screen and the progress of the tube from time to time as I was manipulated on the body bench. Hats off to the doctor who performed this little bit of threading for a fine job. I'm grateful that he didn't miss a turn!

Once the catheter is in position, a solution is injected into the tube and thence joins the blood in the vein, while X rays are simultaneously taken, tracing the path of the solution into the vessels that feed the heart. The subsequent X-ray film shows whether blockage of the blood vessels to the heart exists, and, if so, *where*. It is when the solution, whatever it is called, is injected into the vein and then comes into contact with the blood that a reaction takes place, and this reaction consists of a very warm sensation, which engulfs the body and is accompanied by a feeling of nausea subject to regurgitation. Even though this passes quickly, the unfortunate part of this test is that often it must be repeated several times until the doctor in charge is satisfied that the test has produced the results necessary for complete evaluation of any heart damage that may have occurred during the initial heart attack. The results of these tests are used to determine the future care that should be extended. Again, if you have had the test, you know what it is like; if you have not but know you will have the test, don't worry—no pain at all, only a little discomfort. On the following day, July 10, 1975, I was discharged from the hospital with a two-week follow-up appointment scheduled with my doctor to discuss my total condition and future course of action.

I had survived! We have survived! You and I have undergone a heart attack, suffered the immediate effects of it, and have, with the help of many people, lived to look back on a hair-tingling experience and hopefully forward to many years of reasonably good health and productivity. God has been with us—who can be against us?

DECISION FOR
OPEN-HEART SURGERY

For two weeks after my discharge from the hospital, I confess that I did little or nothing in terms of any physical activity except to enjoy the luxury of my own chair and the pampered spoiling of my family in terms of my wishes and desires. I did exercise as directed and improved on a daily basis until I felt, at least from a mental point of view, as well as I had before my heart attack.

The days passed swiftly and the date arrived for my scheduled appointment with the doctor to discuss the results of the diagnostic tests I had undergone prior to being sent home; the doctor and I would also discuss a future course of action predicated on the results of the tests as determined by a team of coronary specialists. What I had was simple: arteriosclerotic cardiovascular disease, coronary sclerosis with acute myocardial infarction (a heart attack). What was to be recommended was still a mystery.

I would be less than honest if I did not say that both my wife and I were apprehensive when we arrived at the hospital for my appointment. In the back of our minds, I imagine we had thought about the possibility of my needing surgery, but at the same time had hoped that the amount of damage done to my heart during the attack had been slight and that medication and a watchful eye over strenuous physical work might be the answer.

Our questions were answered during the next few minutes as we were ushered in to discuss the total situation with the doctor in charge of my case. In a very controlled and efficient manner, he explained that the lower portion of my heart had been irrevocably damaged by the heart attack. He also indicated that the heart had an amazing capacity to overcome and to compensate for a given deficiency, and that anything that could be done to complement that capacity would be a plus factor in terms of my total longevity. The heart catheterization film showed clearly that one of the vessels feeding the heart was blocked and it was the correction of this blockage that posed the question at hand. Very carefully, the doctor explained the history of open-heart surgery at La Crosse Lutheran Hospital, the records that had been documented on all previous cases, the total number of such surgical procedures, the percentage of success and failures, the implications of age in conjunction with surgery, the overall physical condition of the patient and its relation to success, the theoretical advantage of additional years of life (which such a successful surgical procedure produced), and the theoretical number of years of life projected without surgery. All in all, the doctor spelled out, in general terms, the pros and cons of bypass surgery in as simple and plain a way as he possibly could. He even wrote out for me on a piece of paper the mathematical possibility of living to certain age brackets with and without surgery, his figures predicated on medical records compiled to that date by the hospital. It was apparent that the course of surgery was theoretically the most advantageous in terms of overall outlook. Granted, one could die on the operating table—but then an accident could happen anywhere at any time and a life could be snuffed out.

If you have had this kind of decision to make, I know that you did not find the answer simple, and neither did I. My wife, of course, was present during this meeting, but other than asking questions of the doctor to help clarify the explanations, she did not attempt to influence my decision in any way. Whatever decision was to be made, I was to make it.

Continued discussion about the surgery itself prompted the following remarks. The surgical procedure would involve opening the chest cavity and then locating the obstructed blood vessel to the heart. Once the obstructed blood vessel was located, the patient would be placed on the artificial heart pump; the heart itself would be therefore bypassed and relieved temporarily of its primary function. I can remember asking the doctor what would happen to the heart if it was bypassed and drained of blood—would it stop? The doctor explained that the heart would be deflated without a complete supply of blood, but would continue to beat, but in a fashion that would allow the surgeon to work with much greater ease and precision than would be possible if the heart were functioning at its primary level. During the time when the heart was bypassed, a blood vessel of sound construction and internal clarity would be selected from the chest area, if appropriate, or from the right or left leg if that was more appropriate. This vessel would then be surgically fastened to the obstructed vessel prior to and following the obstruction, thereby creating what was commonly known as a bypass to correct the deficient supply of blood. The doctor in charge of this surgery would be Doctor A. Erik Gundersen, Chief of Cardiac Surgery, La Crosse Lutheran Hospital. I was told that Dr. Gundersen would meet with me prior to the surgery to answer any questions that I might have.

At this time I was prompted to ask the question that I, and other heart attack victims, had asked a thousand times— why me? I had always heard that the possibility of a heart attack happening to a thin person was very unlikely, and at one hundred and fifty pounds, I could hardly be described as heavy. The response to this question has left me with the feeling that not one but a combination of factors determine whether a person will experience a heart attack during his lifetime. Playing important roles in this regard are the factors of heredity (including metabolism, blood pressure, and related physiological forces), dietary factors unique to our American way of life (high fat and cholesterol foods), and, equally as important, the absence of a daily, planned, and adaptive physical activity program.

As my mother had experienced high blood pressure problems during her lifetime, and as both of my older brothers have experienced heart attacks, heredity must surely have played a role in my attack; and as I have been guilty of being fond of foods containing high amounts of cholesterol, certainly this was a contributing factor. Finally, in regard to exercise, my professional responsibilities as a high school principal entail a minimum amount of physical activity. The seed of my heart attack had been planted and took root in not one but all three of the factors mentioned, and although I could have altered the latter two if not the first, concern unfortunately does not become a reality until misfortune occurs.

It appeared that my questions had been answered, a decision was to be made, and I said "proceed." As there was no point in delay, my doctor indicated that the first open date for surgery was August 20, 1975, and that I should check into the hospital on the 18 of that month for preliminary work and presurgery preparation. The die had been cast—time was now the only intervening factor.

PREPARATION
FOR SURGERY

The two weeks between my decision to have surgery and reporting to the hospital passed uneventfully and all too quickly. I was readmitted to the hospital on August 18, 1975, and welcomed back by the same nurses that had only a few short weeks before seen me discharged from my initial attack.

My personal outlook at this time was very good, and in all honesty I can say that any fears and apprehensions about the upcoming surgery were duly tempered by the visitations of many friends that had personally experienced similar surgery in the past. The reassurance and lay explanations of their experiences helped to counteract any fears that may have been present, and my gratitude is extended to them for their assistance during this period. I am hopeful that the future will allow me the opportunity to meet with and to give reassurance to patients with similar needs in similar ways.

The initial day of my readmittance was uneventful, and time was mostly spent getting organized and relaxed. The second day of my stay was different, however, and was filled with the routine activities of blood tests, urine specimen checks, chest X rays, electrocardiographs, and related tests. Significant about the day was the visitation to my room in a very personal manner by the doctor who was to perform my surgery, Dr. Erik Gundersen. A direct, matter-of-fact man with a very plain manner and with the capacity to relate on a one-to-one basis easily, Dr. Gundersen carefully explained the procedure that he was going to follow during the surgery from chest entry to the finding of the affected vein, to the use of the artificial heart machine, to the selection of the

29

proper replacement vein, the implanting of the replacement vein, and the closure upon completion of the operation. He made every effort to explain all items of concern in a calm and reassuring manner, and was successful in conveying all of the information in a manner that induced a feeling of complete security. He even explained that on the following morning attendants would shave my chest and my legs in preparation for surgery, and that the legs were to be shaven in case it was necessary to secure a vein from a leg to be used in the bypass surgery. If this was not necessary and a vein could be secured from the chest area, the latter approach would be used. The doctor left me with an assurance of well-being and security.

The following morning saw additional blood tests and the shaving promised by the doctor. Not one but two male attendants presented themselves to do the job at hand—one an apparently experienced young man in this art and the second an apprentice. Looking back on this episode, I would not be surprised in the least to find that this shaving experience was planned, at least partially, to take my mind off the surgery of consequence and direct it to the surgery of shaving! The older and apparently more experienced of the two attendants did a beautiful job on my chest and one leg, while the apprentice inflicted so many minor wounds that my one leg looked like a freshly plucked pheasant that had been hit by seventy-six pellets, with each pellet wound oozing blood. I have never heard so many apologies for a bad job well done. This beautiful job of preparation was all I could think about.

When the two attendants finished, some additional blood tests were taken, and at approximately 8:00 A.M. I was wheeled from my room on a mobile cart to the surgical area of the hospital. Thinking back about this moment in time, I can recall no apprehension of any kind, and I am sure that during some of the routine blood tests, a sedative of some type was administered in preparation for surgery, because when the attendant left me on the mobile cart in the hallway,

I was cognizant of many people—doctors and nurses—in the area for a brief time . . . and then, nothing. I had either been administered a sedative that caused me to sleep, or was rendered unconscious by some other means. It was apparently my turn for surgery, and I was not going to be allowed the privilege of watching!

POST SURGERY

The first couple of days that I spent in the intensive care and cardiac care units of the hospital following my bypass surgery were days of just that, intensive care, and I do not recall any specific problems that were encountered. My wife has since informed me that after surgery I was not a sight to behold, as my mechanical attire was more complex than that of my initial stay in intensive care. I can only say that I am grateful that all of the devices used have been perfected to a point where each serves a vital function in the process of recuperation, and recuperate I did. Two days after surgery, I was transferred from the cardiac care unit of the hospital to a private room for the final days of therapy, rejuvenation, and rehabilitation.

I must indicate at this time that the most aggravating thing that I experienced during my post-surgical convalescence and rehabilitation was the extreme ache that I experienced in both shoulders when an effort was made to do any form of exercise involving the movement of my upper body. However, after having my chest completely opened by surgically splitting the sternum and separating the two halves of the rib cage by use of a mechanical separator, it is understandable that the shoulders were forced, of necessity, to a backward position unlike their normal setting! The ache in my shoulders and the tenderness of my chest incision (they used wire stitching to put the sternum back together) were the two most obvious discomforts of my surgery other than a general weakness that time would accommodate.

My care was super and the nurses that took care of me on a daily basis were beautiful in the true sense of the word. The doctors (not one but several) visited me daily, and blood tests, X rays, and inhalation therapy exercises were almost daily and routine activities. I believe there was some concern about the presence of fluid in my lungs for a short period, but the inhalation therapy cleared this up with no ill effects.

From the first day after leaving the cardiac care unit I was subjected to daily physical therapy exercises, which contributed greatly to my overall feeling of well-being. As not only medical care, but time itself enhanced my healing process, so did the exercise contribute to both my physical and mental improvement. Exercises began on the first day with simple movements of the legs and arms; for example, I sat up for meals in a chair and fed myself, rather than having a nurse help me. From this beginning I advanced to walking fifty feet with assistance, first once a day and then twice daily, and then being introduced to standing warmup exercises consisting of full shoulder abductions, holding your arms straight out from the shoulders (this was the most difficult for me), and regular leg abductions while leaning against a wall. Being promoted to bathroom privileges without assistance and sitting in a chair for brief periods between and during meals and at bedtime became goals to meet and overcome, as did adding side bends and torso twists and being allowed the privilege of walking to the floor solarium two times a day.

On about the fifth or sixth day of my convalescence, the physical therapist introduced one-pound weights to my exercise program when shoulder abductions were done, and added knee bends and four-way body bends, forward and backward, to my routine. In addition, we began to walk the length of the hospital corridor and to walk down one flight of stairs, returning by means of the elevator. Each day proved a better one in terms of overall physical condition, while at the same time continuous daily medical checks, blood tests, and periodic chest X rays substantiated my good progress. The last few days of my hospital stay saw my exercises and ward activity schedule at optimum performance, with blood pressure and pulse checks within normal ranges. Two days before I was discharged from the hospital, I was scheduled for a modified graded exercise test (GXT) similar to the one I had taken after my initial heart attack and prior to my discharge from the hospital after that event. This test was completed without incidence and in apparently a satisfactory manner, as the day after the test proved to be my discharge date from the hospital—August 30, 1975.

It's a good feeling to go home, and the happiness I felt at this simple act is hard to explain. My two brothers, both of whom live in the La Crosse area, were at the hospital at the appointed time, one having volunteered to drive our family car with me in it to our home, and the other driving a second car so that they both could return to their homes. I was instructed to stop in the hospital dietary office on my way out for instructions about the low cholesterol diet that the doctor wanted me to follow, and I was also given a printed controlled exercise program and instructed to follow it precisely.

Briefly, the low-cholesterol diet consisted of chicken, turkey, fish and veal often, but no shellfish, fish roe, caviar, organ meats, duck, goose, or mutton. When I purchased meat, I was to buy only lean cuts of beef, lamb, pork, and ham, avoiding heavily marbled meats such as rib roasts, porterhouse steaks, and spareribs. I was also to avoid bacon, sausage, frankfurters, cold cuts, and luncheon meats such as salami and liverwurst, prepared casseroles, frozen dinners, and canned foods with fat content. When I selected vegetables, I could buy fresh, frozen, or canned vegetables without fat. Concerning fruits, I was to buy fresh, frozen, canned or dried fruits. For desserts and breads I was to buy fruit sherbet or sugar candies (without milk chocolate or fat), marshmallows, jellies and jams, avoiding commercial biscuits, muffins, doughnuts, sweet rolls, cakes, rich crackers, egg and cheese bread, cookies, and pies. I was also to avoid mixes for biscuits, muffins, and cakes (except angel food cake). In terms of milk products, I was to buy margarine with liquid corn oil or safflower oil listed as the first ingredient, skim milk, buttermilk, and cheeses made with skim milk and low cholesterol corn oil cheese such as Cheez-ola. I was instructed to read the labels on products, being careful to avoid hydrogenated fat or shortening, butter, cream, egg yolks, whole milk, lard, or coconut oil. In addition, I was to avoid butter, cream, sour cream, whole milk, two-percent milk, and cheeses made with whole milk or cream (cheddar, swiss, blue, cream, etc.). I was also to avoid nondairy substitutes for milk and cream because they usually contain coconut oil. Taboo was also the word with ice cream, commercial puddings, and milk chocolate (cocoa was permissible). The hardest thing for me to take was the fact that I was to have no more than three egg yolks a week, and I feel that if I have broken the diet to any degree of severity, it is in this area. As I have said earlier, the most significant thing about the road to rehabilitation, and more importantly in my mind the road to better health and the avoidance of heart problems, is in the food we eat. The choice is ours—cholesterol or not!

The progressive exercise program that I was to follow was explicit in detail and I imagine somewhat the same in content throughout the country. The important points about the exercise program were walking and regularity of the exercise. Each day I was to do a specific number of warm-up exercises consisting of side bends, knee touches, and waist bends before beginning my walk schedule, which for the first two weeks consisted of progressively increasing my walking distance from one block out and one block back on the first day to ten blocks out and ten blocks back by the fifth day of the program. This walking distance was maintained for the first two weeks of the program, as long as my pulse rate did not exceed 115 beats at the end of each daily walk. The program for the third and fourth week consisted of walking a measured mile out and a measured mile back in a total time of 40 minutes, as long as my pulse rate did not exceed 115 beats at the end of each daily walk. The fifth and sixth week of the exercise program saw the distance increased to a measured mile and one-half in 60 minutes with the same pulse rate conditions, and the seventh and eighth week saw the distance increased to two miles in a total of 72 minutes. Needless to say, the exercises went well, and I was conscientious in my fulfillment of same during the time in question and for the number of weeks indicated prior to my full-time return to work responsibilities. Exercise is a vital link to the maintenance of physical fitness, second only to the dietary needs of daily living.

CONCLUSION

A little over four years have passed since I underwent my heart surgery, and one of the most significant changes personally, other than the fact that I feel fine, is the increase in weight that I have experienced. Prior to my surgery, I weighed one hundred and fifty pounds, and since surgery, abstinence from smoking, and the development of an increased appetite, I am now tipping the scales at one hundred and eighty-five pounds for an increase of appropimately thirty-five pounds.

My general health has been excellent and periodic visits to my doctor for routine examinations has corroborated his fondest hopes for my recovery and resumption of daily activities. Oh, I have had occasions when I have had negative feelings such as a feeling of fullness in the chest, extreme headaches, overtiredness, and shortness of breath; however, I am convinced that it would be easy to blame all of my ills on my heart and so, rather than compound an evil, I have chosen to visit my doctor regularly, exercise when possible, watch my diet, and do those things in general that have been recommended to me as positive ways to get the most mileage from the castle I call my body. With the help of the good Lord, that could be a lot of mileage.

Soon after my discharge from the hospital, I was also given the opportunity to join a La Crosse, Wisconsin based organization known as the "Open Heart Surgery Association." The membership of this group consists of those who have experienced surgery such as mine and many who have experienced heart surgery of a much more delicate nature. These people, along with their spouses, meet not only as a social group to share their experiences and learn from one another, but also as a contributing group to the hospital from whose

facilities their destinies were determined. I have wholeheart-
edly endorsed and maintained membership in this organization, but because of distance and work responsibilities have
not attended meetings and social functions as much as I
would have liked to. I am hopeful that the future will provide
me a greater opportunity to do this. Should you have the
opportunity to join such an organization, do so, as I am sure
you will benefit immensely from your membership. If there
isn't any such organization in your area, start one!

In closing, let me say that I am happy to be alive, and
you should be also. The emergency facilities of a small town,
the physical facilities of emergency vehicles and hospitals, and
the skill and God-given talents of caring people all worked
together to assist me—and many others—through a trying
period. I am now, and forever will be, grateful to all who
helped me in any way. How many years will you and I still
enjoy life? Who knows? Perhaps five, maybe ten, twenty,
thirty, or even more years will be ours to enjoy. The answer
to that question rests in greater hands than ours. Perhaps
it is best said in the ninth chapter of Proverbs, verses eight
to twelve as follows:

> Do not reprove a scoffer, or he will hate you; reprove a
> wise man, and he will love you. Give instructions to a
> wise man, and he will be still wiser; Teach a righteous
> man and he will increase in learning. The fear of the Lord
> is the beginning of wisdom, and the knowledge of the Holy
> One is insight. *For by me your days will be multiplied,
> and years will be added to your life.* If you are wise, you
> are wise for yourself; if you scoff, you alone will bear it.

Time is as important as we want to make it, as full as the
measure we pour. Plan to make your life a full one, predicated on the positive values of living rather than the negative
values of dying.

So you had a heart attack? Well, so did I, and so did
thousands of other men and women just like you and me.
Look up, you've got a long way to go and a lot to do. Let's
both get at it!